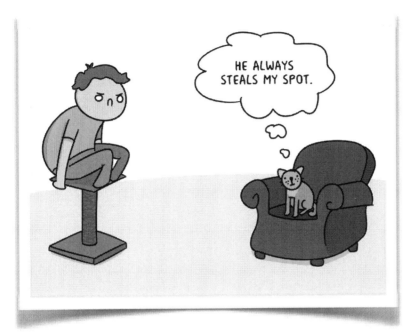

JUST ONE MORE PURR
Chronic and Terminal Illness Support for Cats and the Humans Who Love Them

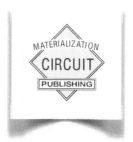

ISBN: 978-1-7753371-2-6

Cover design artwork and book layout by Melanie Dixon. Editing and proofreading by Kim West.

Dixon, Melanie
Just One More Purr / Melanie Dixon.—1st ed.
Visit the author:
https://meldawn.wixsite.com/melaniedawndixon

JUST ONE MORE PURR

Chronic and Terminal Illness Support for Cats and the Humans Who Love Them

MELANIE DIXON

PROTECTIVE BLESSING FOR CATS

Bast of beauty and of grace
Protectress of the feline race
Shield (name of pet) from all hurt and harm
And keep him/her always safe and warm.

Watch over (name of pet) from day to day
And guide him/her home if he/she should stray
And grant him/her much happiness
And a good life free of strife and stress.

From *Everyday Magic: Spells & Rituals for Modern Living*
by Dorothy Morrison

TABLE OF PURRS

Introduction—Just One More Purr

It was bedtime when I was preparing Isabel's food so she wouldn't wake me up in the middle of the night to eat. She came running into the kitchen. "Meow meow meow," she began, releasing a long and endless series of excited meows.

"What's wrong?" I asked, giving her head a good pet.

She gazed up at the counter where her medications were located.

I held up her bottle of Ursodiol, one of the medications that managed her liver disease.

"Drugs? Do you want drugs?"

"Mra!" she declared, then waited patiently.

I quickly grabbed a syringe off the counter—I had them pre-filled for 24 hours in advance—and knelt down, slid the tip into the side of her mouth, then squeezed a tiny stream of fluid into her mouth. Seriously, by now I could do this in the dark.

"Mra!" she said, thanking me. She smugly walked away, now that her job of telling me what to do was done.

"But you know that wasn't the kitty morphine, right?" I held up the bottle of buprenorphine but she ignored me. I jokingly called it "kitty morphine", even though her vet would correct me and say it was not even close.

We developed a symbiotic relationship where she'd communicate her needs to me, and I would interpret them into how I was to care for her. Our wonderful way of communicating allowed me to do a better job as a kitty caregiver.

If you're caring for a sick, chronically ill, or terminally ill cat, you too may develop this instinct of how to care for your cat by what they tell you. They may give off various signals, sounds, or looks that can give you a clue.

And if you still can't figure it out, this book will help you to cope. It also helps to have a great sense of humour, to help you cope when your cat wipes her bum on the wall, or vomits all over the bed at 3 am.

This is a book that covers the long-term stressful effects of caring for a sick, or chronically or terminally ill cat. It's not meant to be all that long, as likely you don't have a lot of time for reading during these stressful moments in life. This is a book for the dedicated cat owner who loves their cat(s), and will do almost anything for them. In fact, you may already have.

My book may help you if your cat is injured or temporarily sick, but since this book is focussed on the stressors of knowing your cat is going to pass, and the mental health challenges associated with that, you may find better advice on cat injury or illness care in other books.

This isn't your average cat care guide that tells you how to look after kitty, from kittenhood to senior years. There are thousands of cat care books out there, cat care by breed, cat first aid, and cat humour books. Instead, this book is about providing the best support and care for your sick cat and you, so that you can continue to live a normal and joyful life. In other words, this book is for your benefit. But if you already have a sick or terminally ill or chronically ill cat, you may already be drowning in fur, or something much worse: kitty bodily fluids.

This book is not meant as a replacement for veterinarian care. I can't stress enough how important it is to take your cat to the vet at the first sign of illness. So, if your cat is chronically or terminally ill, you understand it to mean that your cat is at the vet's clinic several times each year for the best kitty care. This book can't replace these necessary steps.

Nor is this a book to help you decide whether you should euthanize your cat or not. However, there is a chapter at the back on what comes next, should your cat pass naturally, or you decide on euthanasia to ease their journey. Maybe you decide to euthanize, maybe you choose to look after your cat until they naturally pass—it's your choice.

I've also been impartial to religion in this book. Many people from different faiths may believe in a kitty heaven, or a human heaven where our beloved pets wait for us. I have written this book to be inclusive of everyone—in every country, religion, gender, and belief system—because we all love our cats more than anything. You may find more info online about cat prayers, if you wish.

This book also involves nonjudgemental advice about cats. Whether your cat is indoors, outdoors, or a combination of both, that doesn't matter here. As long as you care, that's all that matters.

That's why this book is for the living. You have a sick cat, and you're stressed out of your mind. You miss sleep, feel sick to the stomach, and may even have been yelled at at work for being late or unproductive—it's happened to me.

You may suffer depression from your cat being sick. You may have found that all the joy is gone from your life. You've gone from the happy days of when you initially adopted your kitten or cat, to a life of stress. The bills are piling up, you feel awful. Perhaps your health condition is flaring up, costing you money. Your cat is crying all hours of the day and night, and scratches and bites when you attempt care.

This book isn't about how to pay for vet bills or cat care supplies either. If you do need help, you can ask family or friends for help, seek the services of a low-cost SPCA vet, use your credit cards, cash in a savings account or RRSP, get a loan, or set up a GoFundMe account. There are even loan companies that focus on pet care loans.

Now you begin to understand the need for this book. It's full of wisdom for those committed cat owners who must live one day at a time. We'll also inject some humour into it, because caring for cats is often fun, even when they're not cooperative.

Yes, this book is for the living, because the day you adopted your loving cat you made a commitment to look after him/her for the rest of their life, through the good times and the bad. But, most of all, you love Fluffy, Tigger, Isabel, Monty, Your Cat's Name Here, and that's what's most important of all.

There is advice in this book about how to better look after your cat. You can imagine there's a big disconnect between being at the clinic where your vet is telling you to give kitty some medication, how the feeding tube works, or how to give injections, and the time you bring kitty home. Somehow, they never tell you what it's really like looking after a sick pet.

It can be even worse looking after a sick pet than it can be to look after a sick spouse or a sick child, or elderly parents. There are special challenges to looking after a pet cat. A cat doesn't understand why you're poking and prodding them and making them do all these hateful things—poking needles into their skin, forcing food and meds into their mouth, sticking an IV into their leg. And, they may hate you for it and hide. A cat also cannot tell you that they're feeling sick, or they have pain somewhere in their body, that they have itchy skin, or that they have blurred vision or feel dizzy.

In less than a few hours you'll gain the tools for surviving, with an outcome that's less stressful. You'll be better able to care for your pet, to become happier, calmer, and more positive.

I've put in the time searching for answers, so there's no need for you to spend hours searching for the information you need when it's all right here. The tools and advice you need is right within this book.

Some of the chapters may overlap with each other, but it's always good to have positive advice drilled into your head.

Finally, this book is designed to help you to get through this rough patch in life. It could be a temporary situation. It may be for years—my own cat Isabel had been suffering from liver disease for over two years before she passed away.

This is a gimmick-free book. There are no magic potions or spells to help your cat get better, though if you find they calm you, by all means continue your practices. Likewise, there is no advice on a magical prescription that will cure your pet.

Grab a nice hot drink, and please keep on reading. We're in the fur together.

I Volunteer As Tribute

1. Life Is Meowsome—Finding Isabel

Life should be meowsome, otherwise, there's no point to it. We must get past our challenges. Yes, there is the bad, and there is the good. We must create balance.

My entire life I had cats, except for an extremely long 14 years of renting apartments. Instead, I'd accumulate a large collection of cat ornaments, cat stuffies, and other cat-related objects.

In 2004 I adopted a tabby I named Cristobel. She was fine for most of the years I had her. This was my first experience with a terminally ill cat. In the spring of 2009, the unthinkable happened. For the past year she had rapidly declined, until I learned she had lymphoma, a deadly form of cancer. By the time we knew, she was already in her final days.

I had become so attached to her in only five short years. I was devastated by her vet bills on my part-time income, and totally devastated in my heart. I knew I would adopt another cat one day, I just didn't know when.

Several months passed. I graduated from college as a Medical Office Assistant and First Aid Level Two Attendant, and found a better job. Not a day went by that I did not think of her. My boyfriend, Tiemen, drove me around to all the local shelters. I viewed hundreds of cats, but in my heart none of them were as special to me as Cristobel had been.

"Leave the carrier in the car," I told Tiemen, at Katie's Place Cat Shelter in Maple Ridge, BC, in November 2009. "I won't find a cat here either." He didn't listen to me and brought the pet taxi inside anyway.

We spent two hours looking at cats. I wanted one around two years old, so I would have her for a long time. The staff helped me narrow down the cats that I had seen online. They didn't think a young tabby that looked exactly like Cristobel was the right cat for me, so the hunt continued. They weren't going to let me leave without a cat in that pet taxi either.

At the shelter, I was discouraged; none of the cats really stood out for me. I knew I wouldn't find one here. The hunt for a cat would continue. I was taking this adoption seriously, and we had to be right for each other.

Finally, I decided to look at the older cats. There was nothing else to do on that day but go home anyway. I looked at 50 more, even the ones in the quarantine room.

I entered what must have been the last room of the shelter. All these cats were older, around 6 or more years. Not the right age, but I was just looking.

And then I turned and I saw a gorgeous black, brown and peach tabby! She had the sweetest expression on her face as I stroked her. She had the softest fur, her ears were rounded, and she seemed quite gentle. Her whiskers swooped downward, and she had a wide chest. She kept on looking at me with this creepy smug expression on her face. She looked at me as if to say, "You are my human!"

This was the cat I had been waiting for months to adopt! She looked like an Isabel to me, so I changed her first name of

Cherub to her middle name. We brought her home and she cuddled up to me on that first night, purring contentedly. And she spent the next eight years happy and content, always by my side.

Usually there is an intensive process required for adopting a cat, but with both Cristobel and Isabel, it was sped up so I could bring take home immediately.

Over the years she'd get the same mysterious illness. The routine was the same—take her to the vet—get antibiotics, bring her home and she'd be fine in two weeks' time. In 2012, we had a confirmed diagnosis of pancreatitis. Things went well until March 2015. Isabel started losing large clumps of fur. At first I thought it was simply due to the lovely warm weather we'd been having. But then she began to slowly decline. In April she went into the vet. She was extremely sick this time. I was told it was another episode of pancreatitis.

The next two months were tough. I thought I was going to lose her for sure. Even the vet told me that euthanasia was an option, but I remembered how devastated I was when I did that for Cristobel, so I wouldn't consider that option.

To my surprise, Isabel hung in there for another month. I think we truly kept each other going. One day I thought I'd pop into the vet's clinic to get her some more special prescription diet kitty food. I walked the three blocks to the clinic only to find the doors barred shut. The clinic was gone! Apparently the veterinary business went bankrupt, so what to do now?

There was actually another vet clinic around the corner, so I made an appointment. There, the vet properly diagnosed Isabel with hepatitis, hepatic lipidosis, cholangitis, and pancreatitis. She didn't have triaditis, which involves the bowels, fortunately. Isabel had notable signs of jaundice in her skin and fur.

We finally got Isabel on a good medication plan that cost me over $300 per month, and another $100 per month of special food. This was after I had quit a stressful job I'd had at a medical software company that treated their employees like Apple factory slaves, and did not understand the stress and insomnia I was experiencing at having a sick pet. Since then I've been working as an independent writer and online marketer, but fortunately had some savings to rely on.

I had reached the point where I was tired of feeling stressed out, and even one time became as sick as my cat, as each day was rushed and stressful, with no sleep, and a bundle of cat-related chores to do. I felt that there had to be a better way to cope, perhaps by better managing her healthcare.

With the assistance of Isabel's new vet, we got her stabilized. Isabel had certain challenges where she was in pain from upset tummy, then she'd vomit up more than you'd ever think a small kitty could ever hold in her stomach. I even considered packaging up her vomit and selling it to a jeans brand so it could quickly wear holes in pants for that latest torn-jeans fashion fad. Isabel went from a twelve-pound cat down to under five pounds over the course of two years.

So, what did I do to get through the chaos? I did plenty of research, reading, and searching the internet and the local library. I talked to other pet owners who had chronically or terminally ill pets. I took online seminars and workshops. I even had my MOA—Medical Office Assistant, First Aid Level II, and Pet First Aid certificates and diplomas to back me up.

Why did I do all this for my cat? To survive. It was time for me to learn how to cope, so I could be "present" for her when she was sick.

So, now almost three years have passed. She passed away on September 10, 2017. Once again, I was devastated by the loss of my second cat.

We do not know what caused her liver disease and likely never will. Antibiotics are ineffective. This is the type of mysterious liver disease that a cat sometimes gets. Perhaps she was exposed to poison when she was younger. Perhaps it's hereditary or simply old age. If only it were as simple as diabetes, thyroid disease, or a bacterial or viral infection. But it was none of those things.

As I began to do research, one thing was shockingly clear. Cats are generally euthanized after a liver disease diagnosis, as it quickly leads to death. I was one of the rare ones who decided to try to save her. A friend of mine said I should be proud—how I made her so happy and comfortable in her final years of life.

So, we're back to this point of this book. The first year was tough. One day I acted like a cat and pawed a glass off the countertop. It certainly felt good to release my anger that way, but I couldn't afford to replace my glass! Then I realized that I had to get my feelings under control as my kitty was relying on me for living.

I'm sure that not many people will make this revelation, and it's embarrassing. But it does happen, and I just want you to know that anger is normal.

Anyway, enough about me and my cats. It's now time for you to worry less about your sick, injured, or terminally ill cat, and more effectively look after her and yourself so you have a meowsome life together!

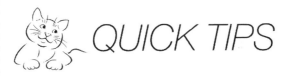

QUICK TIPS

- Remember that life is meowsome.

- You and your cat were meant to be together.

- Learn how to look after your cat.

- The more you know, the better you can live.

2. Platitudes, Catitudes—The Myths of Cat Care

If you have family or friends who've never looked after a sick pet, they don't really know what it's like. At first you're worried because your cat is sick. You book an appointment with the vet and your hope increases. They're going to pull through! That's your typical scenario for when most pets get sick. They're just like us and they do get better.

Then, for a smaller percentage of cats, they acquire long-term, permanent, or terminal illnesses. Often it begins with them not eating their food, requiring a visit to the vet. The vet may not be certain what is wrong. The lab tests are a bit abnormal but perhaps it's nothing. You bring your cat back home. Then on a regular basis, your cat keeps on getting sick until it's like a routine.

Finally, your vet works out that your cat has kidney failure, liver failure, or cancer. Your vet may be hesitant to offer this kind of diagnosis; after all, euthanasia may then be brought up next. Most vets do not want to have to euthanize a pet before their time.

Eventually, you could get a diagnosis that doesn't make you happy. You may wonder how you'll cope, as likely kitty will need some extra care that comes out of your day, and also your pocketbook.

You may even get the prognosis that your cat needs palliative care—the process where a cat is simply made to be as comfortable as possible while they live out their last days with their beloved owner.

Where you may be experiencing challenges in looking after your sick kitty may come from people who really have no idea what you're going through—the turmoil and emotions in your mind that your cat is going to die and leave you all alone—there, we said it. You get the gist of the problem right here.

Most of us who have sick pets just do it—we look after them until the end—because they're our family. You're your cat's own expert. You already know what makes them happy, their unique schedule, and how to look after them.

The last thing you need to hear are platitudes from friends or family. "He'll get better." "It'll turn out all right." "She doesn't look all that sick." But you just smile and nod your head.

What's even worse when you're looking after a sick kitty is when you hear stupid advice from people who are supposedly your closest friends and family. This is advice from people who don't have a clue what you're going through.

You can offer some humorous retorts to help you deal with the situation, but only you may find them funny.

One of the first you'll hear is to euthanize your cat. You can always get another one. *Sure,* you think, *hop in the car with me. I need another friend.*

The next one isn't so extreme, but they may suggest that you give up your cat, like she's some sort of disposable rag doll. *Great,* you may be thinking, *why doesn't your husband hop in the car and I'll drop him off at the shelter too?*

Some people may think you're being petty when there are worse things wrong with the world. You can politely remind them of that time when you listened to their complaints. You must explain that your cat is a member of your family. By now you've likely won the pot because you've collected a fine hand of useless comments!

You're probably going to have to bite your tongue a lot and smile and thank people for their advice. But always remember, Tigger is your cat, so never let anyone tell you what to do with your own pet's medical care.

There is no timetable for a sick cat who's on their great journey. Some cats live to 19 years old and beyond with health conditions. Your vet may give you a timeframe or you may look up info online, but just ignore that type of advice.

A few other issues you may have with people could involve a lack of support from those closest to you. You may have to come clean if you've been hiding your cat's illness from everyone. You need to let people know that you need their help and support.

Often a parent is the one responsible for kitty care while the kids barely even do anything. Often this is your fault, not theirs. The kids do want to help out, so assign small tasks for them to do, such as ensuring the cat's water bowl is clean, the crunchies are topped up, brushing their fur, or scooping the poop.

If you have an unsupportive spouse, you're going to have some big problems. Chances are you have other issues in your relationship. And this is the worst time to get through it. In this instance, counselling may benefit. But if you're biding your time, try to get through it as you need those vet bills covered!

Another problem may be with work or unsupportive bosses. Even if kitty keeps you up all night, you still have to go to work the next day. I suggest that you carry on with your routine as much as possible, rather than calling in a sick day. You'd be surprised at how much better you feel when you're on a regular routine.

For myself, I soon learned how to live on only five or six hours a night of sleep. And remember, it's temporary until you get kitty stabilized and sleeping through the night. In fact, it can be rather fun staying up all night with your cat, partying and having fun—well, almost!

Many people in your life may hold firm to the myths of cat care. But you're one step ahead of them. You've accepted your challenge of looking after kitty, and you'll do everything it takes to ensure that you both have a wonderful life together, even if it's only for a few more purrs.

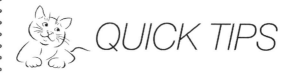 *QUICK TIPS*

- Be immune to stupid platitudes.

- Your cat is a beloved family member.

- Maintain your sense of humour.

- Enjoy each and every purr.

3. Welcome to the Mew World—Creating a Royal Care Plan

This is the new normal, your new identity, your new relationship with your cat. It'll also be a new one for friends and family. You'll make new friends. You'll gain a new sense of purpose. When you have an ailing cat you'll also have ample opportunity to bond further with them.

No one will tell you these secrets, not even the vet. You'll find out for yourself. It's a lot like looking after a sick child. You'll become extremely tired, even mentally. This is due to the extra time and care of feeding your pet, giving them treatments and medications, and taking extra time in cleaning up the messes they make.

It'll also take extra time spent in comforting your pet, shopping for special products to make them feel comfortable, and taking time to make them items that you can't find in the store. You'll also need to set aside extra time to take your cat to the vet, or transport them to a cat sitter.

You're going to lose sleep at night, through anxiety and worry, and even perhaps because kitty is crying and howling. I live in a small apartment where I couldn't lock Isabel into a basement when she was unwell. Not that I advise you doing that.

Your body will adjust and expect insomnia. Your hair and nails will grow thinner. If you have a disease or health condition, it will worsen by 50%. I suddenly developed a case of bad eczema on my elbows. I was fortunate it wasn't on my face. My stomach was upset after every meal, and I had internal pain, as if I had a psychosomatic illness right along with my cat.

You'll experience anxiety and anger about all of these things and more. You'll worry about not being able to pay your rent or mortgage, or buy yourself food, because all your money is going to your pet.

You'll also arrive home from work with a new sense of purpose. You'll look forward to seeing your cat. Now you can comfort her as you relax in front of the TV. If she shows interest in your dinner, then that's a good sign! (But don't give any of it to her!)

Here are 6 tips on how to create a royal care plan for you and your cat.

I. Set a New Routine

Our cats love to tell us what to do, from when they first want their food in the morning, to when it's time to go to bed at night.

There's going to be change in your routine for when you must adjust to their illness or disease. The trick is to make them think it was their idea first.

My cat would come running when I said "brush" or "you're missing out". If you can establish some sort of routine for giving them their food and their medications that can shorten the experience by even five minutes, that's extra time to do all the other things.

Why did my cat run to, "you're missing out"? It's just something I started saying to her at bedtime. But maybe she understood? Who knows.

Her routine was fairly active between 6 am and noon, whereupon she'd demand first, second, and third breakfasts. This was good because she had an anorexic body and was allowed to eat as much as she wanted.

Then I'd give her the first round of meds. I'd wash up and get on with my day, which was working from home writing, doing social media for clients, graphic design, working on websites, and doing business smackdowns—also known as helping businesses analyze why the customers aren't buying.

Isabel would get up once or twice during the day for a bite to eat. Around my dinner time was generally her dinnertime. Then she'd go back to bed.

Around 9 pm she'd get up and tell me it was time for her last round of meds. This was also when she'd get three fresh glasses and bowls of water around her home.

Then, we'd snuggle up in bed together and read. Or, she slept. Then we'd do it all over again the next day.

On the weekends she'd get special care, such as clawsy clippin's, a washcloth rubdown, face and butt cleaning, food station cleaning, or anything else that needed to be done.

You'll want to stick to the same routine each day as it eases the burden of giving meds, cleaning the cat box and cat dishes, and spending time looking after your cat. Your cat will be less likely to hide during these times. Remember my story in the introduction about giving my cat her drugs, and how, if I was late, she'd remind me?

II. Keeping the Mind Active and Alert Through Play

Even though Isabel didn't play with her toys anymore, she still showed an interest in the world surrounding her. She loved to look at bugs, and cars driving past on the street. Sometimes she'd grab one of my things: yarn or a necklace.

If she did play, we'd play together. I'd toss a ribbon around, and she'd bat at it once or twice. I could still see the kitten in her, even if she didn't get up and run around.

Some other things we did included allowing her out into the hallway. This seemed to fascinate her. One time I picked her up and carried her to the mailbox. When we got back to my apartment she wanted to do it again.

I think it's important to do some little things that provide interest for your cat on a daily basis, as she's still alive, and you want to give her the encouragement and let her know that life is still worth living, even when you're a geriatric kitty.

Even though your cat may not play as much as they did as a kitten, it's still important to entertain and keep their mind active. Place a few of their favourite toys in their kitty care station. You may have to encourage them to play by moving that mousie around. Sometimes they simply love to watch you play rather than participating. But if they are interested, do encourage them. Sometimes they may simply lie in their beds and provide the occasional swat to that ribbon toy.

Let them watch a cat app on your mobile smart device or laptop computer. Cats like to watch TV shows too.

III. Setting Up a Kitty Care Station

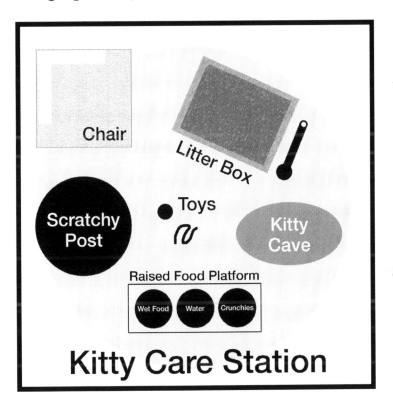

My single most important cat care trick is the following. Check out the illustration. You need to designate a kitty care station in your home. Your cat may be like mine, who could barely walk across the room in her last two weeks. That means doing some interior redecorating of your space.

Most people don't use their dining room space. Set up a space of four feet by four feet. This is solely for the use of your pet. If you have small children, babies, or other pets, you'll need to work out a way to keep them away from this space. Perhaps a room with a door, or a closet that has a door that shuts. If you're worried about kitty hiding under the bed, you can set up walls with cheap cardboard from the grocery store. But often you'll find that kitty is simply too weak and tired, at least in the early days of their illness, to fight you. And if they're on painkillers, it's even better to have a designated space, as it makes cat care a whole lot simpler.

You may also consider noise when choosing the perfect kitty care station. If you have a busy family, the living room or kitchen may not be the best spot to keep your cat. You'll want to minimize noise and activity around your cat. As he nears the end of his life you'll want a happy and soothing environment for him.

On the other hand, a cat may enjoy simply curling up in her kitty cave, knowing that her humans are nearby. If you have a spare room, you may wish to move her station into there for the times when you're entertaining, and have a lot of company over. But do leave the door slightly ajar in case she shows interest in visiting.

While some light classical music can lift the mood of your cat, don't play it for endless hours. Simply play one album for its full length, then turn off the device.

In my kitty care space I'd set it up based on a plus symbol +. If we consider a north, south, east, and west type of layout, set up a freshly scrubbed box with fresh litter to the north. To the south will be placed kitty's wet and dry food bowls, and a water dish. Keep these clean and filled at all times. Again, if you have other pets, you need to keep them away. To the west, set up a soft kitty bed or chair for your pet. To the east, set up a kitty cave where kitty can hide. This will provide a comforting cocoon for them to go when they're not feeling well. Their toys will fit in the middle.

Beneath your pet's possessions place a washable mat or a large towel. This should be something that you can toss in the washing machine at least once a day. It's useful to purchase more than one towel. Use old towels, or even old bath mats. If your cat can't aim properly in the box then you can place a plastic tarp beneath.

If your cat has trouble jumping up, you're going to have to place the high kitty perches into storage. The last thing you want is for your cat to fall from a high location and break a bone. You may have to discourage her from jumping onto window sills or other tall furniture. You can move it out of her room, or block it with boxes or other furniture.

There are special carpeted steps that you can buy for your dogs to help them up onto your bed. A cat can use these too. Some are basic plastic, and some are covered in carpet. Buy what you can afford.

It also helps to buy large foam tiles—found at any big-box

department store in the kids' section—and place them around your cat's living space. This provides a soft place to walk, and if they still use their shorter scratchy posts, it provides a nice soft pad to land on, rather than hardwood flooring.

You can also do all this and still have your kitty try to jump up to sleep on the couch. I suggest placing a soft washable towel or cloth where she likes to sleep, and soft foam tiles or cushions directly beneath, in case she falls off. You may need to assist your pet on and off furniture.

Place a clean, but super-soft washable pillow in their kitty bed. This provides an additional level of comfort. There are also special cat heating pads that you can buy from your local pet shop. These are tested for pet safety and have auto shut-offs, in case you forget to turn it off when you go to bed.

These heating pads maintain the perfect temperature for your cat to enjoy. As cats get older or get sick, their bodies have trouble maintaining a good body temperature. Human heating pads don't work as well. I tried one for Isabel, and it was a lot of work maintaining a proper temperature level, or remembering to turn it off. I advise you get one just for your pet. A pet heating pad is also safe in case they pee in their beds. The cover can be removed and washed.

Remember to wash your kitty's linens at least once per week. This keeps them clean and fresh-smelling for everyone, and is also sanitary for a time when kitty's immune system may not be as strong as when she was a kitten.

The lighting levels of a room can be kept at regular day or

nighttime lighting, but when the humans are asleep, give her eyes a break and turn off all the lights.

You should be aware that even healthy cats can be affected by eating houseplants, human foods, and flowers, and be affected by fragrances and scents. Candles, essential oils, and aromatherapy devices can also be harmful. There is new information online that states that even the most natural essential oils can be harmful for cats.

What you can use instead of essential oils is a product called Feliway. This is a synthetic copy that is similar to your cat's facial pheromones. It helps to keep your cat feeling they're in a secure and safe territorial environment.

Sick kitties can be even more affected by scented products in the home, and it can lead to additional toxicities building up in their bodies. Remove all houseplants, flowers, candles, air fresheners, and other scented products from your cat's space.

Never feed them human foods. And, ensure you wash your hands before touching your cat. If your cat likes to lick your hands or arms, this is especially important. If you need a hand moisturizer, use a dry kitty shampoo—it's surprisingly moisturizing.

There can also be other hazards, such as from Christmas trees, balloons, ribbon, small children's toys, jewellery, and craft supplies. Keep an eye on your cat during holiday celebrations, and dispose of garbage ASAP.

This may all seem like a lot of information to take in, and

a lot of work, but with a bit of effort, you should be able to enjoy life, with plenty of purring, for your remaining time together.

IV. Basic Cat Hygiene

When your cat gets older or she feels too sick to clean herself, her fur is going to start getting greasy, and she's going to smell bad. Her bottom may be particularly revolting. Now it's up to you to look after her.

You can purchase dry shampoo for cats, or cat wipes, just in case you need to wipe them down. You can also buy a 100% cotton washcloth and towel, if you don't want to toss wipes in the garbage. Cats often need a bit of help in cleaning out their ears. You can buy specific ear cleansers, or simply use plain water on a cotton puff to clean them out.

Their eyes and noses can get crusties and mucous that gently needs to be wiped off. Do check their nostrils—Isabel would get hardened crust over her nostrils and I'd actually have to use the tweezers to pull it out. This can affect their breathing, so do check to be sure they can breathe well.

Also take a look at their teeth and gums. While most vets don't recommend teeth cleaning when a cat is in her last stages of life, if they're in extreme pain or have a loose tooth, it's something that will have to be dealt with quickly.

V. Where's the Drugs?

Your vet will prescribe medications for your cat. You'll get them in a small white paper bag. You'll have to give all these medications to your cat, three times a day. You get it home, and then, it's like *what the…? But I have to work? My cat sleeps all day…* This is where you become the pet caregiver. It's time to do a rundown of all meds with your vet. If you get confused and can't read the labels, call the vet clinic and ask for a refresher.

It's also 100% important to NEVER give your cat human medications or dog medications from the medicine cabinet. You may be trying to save money, but instead, it'll cost you a very expensive vet bill when your cat has an adverse reaction, or worse.

When you do get your veterinarian-prescribed prescriptions for your cat, it's important to store them in a dry and dark cupboard, away from them, away from children, and away from other pets.

Here are a few tips to consider when giving medications to your cat.

- Is there a better format of medication to give a cat? I had all of Isabel's medications in a flavour-free liquid format that was administered to her through an oral syringe. Flavour-free, because I didn't want to turn her off her food. Your vet can provide medication in liquid format or you can have your vet call in a prescription to a local compounding pharmacy in your city. There are even medications that you simply dab on their ears or skin.

- Can you give her the medication first thing in the morning and in the early evening instead, about 12 hours apart? It's a lot simpler remembering to give your cat her meds first thing in the morning, and first thing when you get home from work.

- There are cat pill poppers that make it easier to pop those pills down their throats. There are smaller pill poppers meant specifically for cats and not dogs, that you can buy online.

- You can buy pill pockets where you can hide their pills. There are also pill pastes that you can wrap around the pill. Some cats may be fooled, while others will spit out the meds.

- There are restraint jackets or suits you can buy for a cat that freaks out when you try to give them medication, or when you need to wipe their fur down. They're like wrapping a towel around your cat but instead you slip it around your cat and click the fasteners or velcro together. Now kitty is restrained and can't scratch you. But watch out for those teeth!

- You can also wrap your cat up in a towel, which works for at least five minutes, which is time enough to administer medication, wipe their eyes and ears down, clean their whiskers and butt, and ensure there are no crusties in their nose that can affect their breathing.

- Some people also like to buy a baby outfit and put their cat in it so they can more easily do cat care. It'll make for some funny photos too—just don't show them to your cat!

- You can also use a harness, but you'll have to tie it around something. You can have a family member gently hold the pet down or stroke her while you're providing care.

- Avoid giving medication with food, as it can create an aversion for their food. The last thing you want is for your cat to stop eating. But if you give your cat a pill orally, or with a medicine dropper, then you can reward them with a treat immediately afterwards.

It's important to offer input to your vet when you are ordering medications. There are many compounding pharmacies that can convert your cat's humongous pills into a liquid format. Ask your vet how to use a syringe to give liquid medication to your cat, or find out if they sell pill pockets or pastes.

Remember to stay calm when you're giving medication to your cat. They can sense our moods and be adversely affected. Put a smile on your face and think happy thoughts. This will help them avoid feeling anxious or fearful.

Now, your life just got simpler and your cat will still love you!

VI. Supervised Feeding

You may have noticed in the Kitty Care Station that there are food dishes which are raised up off the ground. The bowls are also wide and have low rims. This is so your cat isn' annoyed when their whiskers touch the side of the plate. You can buy these bowls from pet supply stores.

I liked to have Isabel's bowls, dishes, and water dishes raised up off the ground. This was so she could sit on the ground and eat more comfortably. There was also a second reason—since she had liver disease, her body produced too much stomach acid. By eating in a more upright position, this kept the stomach acid in her tummy, rather than climbing up into her throat.

For cats who suffer stomach acid or upset stomach, raised bowls also keep stomach acids from travelling up their esophaguses.

Using raised and flat dishes or plates will also avoid whisker stress, which some cats can get. This can discourage them from eating, and that's the last thing you need when your cat already is suffering an upset tummy from their health condition.

My cat was a fussy and picky eater. I had to do everything I could to get her to eat.

Isabel and I had an understanding during those times

when she'd completely stop eating. I'd put her on the counter on top of a towel. I'd then wrap a small towel around her, much like a bib. This meant it was kitty-care time. She was good for at least five minutes, and would stay put.

Sometimes you can train your cat with a similar routine. If not, bundle her up as a kitty purrito, and keep your treatment sessions as short as possible. Oh, and you'll also want to wear an apron, as force feeding can get messy!

You may have to syringe feed your cat with wet cat food and water. When Isabel was at her sickest, the vet said I had to do this SIX TIMES A DAY. But don't worry, once you can encourage your cat to eat, you may have to do it only two or three times a day. As I said earlier, set up a routine in your calendar.

Your vet will have small or large syringes (without the needles on the end) for feeding. These are also called medicine droppers. You can also buy ones with the bulbous rubber end. I've tried them all and prefer to use the middle-sized ones. You'll have to figure out what works best for you.

There are some different canned foods to encourage cats to keep on eating, because if they don't, they can suffer from hepatic lipidosis, which is fatal. The vet doesn't tell you this, but when the liver fails, it can't adequately produce an enzyme that neutralizes ammonia in the blood. Over time, this can affect the brain and cause seizures. Eventually, one big seizure can cause cardiac arrest, then it's time to say goodbye.

This is why force feeding is the single most important

thing to do for your cat when they don't feel well enough to eat. Yes, they may vomit up the food and water afterwards, but I discovered that Isabel would mostly keep it down.

I was frustrated when she wouldn't eat. Then, my vet gave me a food called "Recovery". She took a sniff of what I had in her bowl, ready to suck up into the syringe, and she started eating it. Success! I still had to syringe feed her for a few weeks after that, but she loved the food so much she always gobbled it up.

I also had Isabel on a high-protein-and-fat Royal Canin dry food for kittens. Even though this type of diet isn't ideal for cats in the beginning stages of liver disease, it's best to first find foods that your cat will eat, then go from there.

You should know, if you're doing palliative care for your beloved cat, that ANY CAT FOOD SHE WILL EAT IS GOOD. You've reached the point where a special diet doesn't matter anymore.

Here are a few feeding tips for your kitty.

• Get her to eat.

• Give him foods he enjoys.

• Give her several kitty treats if she likes them.

• Give him chicken, not cooked in any oils or herbs or spices, as a treat too.

- Avoid giving your cat human or dog foods. You still have to avoid toxicity.

- Give your cat a mix of dry and wet food. Mix it up.

- Add a bit of warm water to your cat's food to help body hydration.

- Warm their wet food up in the microwave.

- Buy smaller crunchies, such as those meant for kittens.

- Mash or cut up food if it has large chunks.

- Give fresh lukewarm water twice a day.

- Use filtered water rather than tap water.

- Do not use bottled water as it contains high levels of plastics and toxins.

- Use a medicine dropper or syringe to give water if he's not drinking enough.

- Ask your vet for assistance if nothing else works.

Keep on trying to find foods that are delicious for your cat if she does stop eating. There is something out there just for her.

As Isabel's liver condition progressed, she'd have her periods of not wanting to eat. I'd put her on a mat on the counter and wrap the towel around her. But instead of syringe feeding, I'd spoon feed her. You may discover that your cat loves to eat this way. It helps to encourage them to eat, and it's much simpler than syringe feeding—which can be extremely messy.

But instead of using a regular metal spoon, I went out and bought baby spoons. Not only are these smaller for smaller mouths, but they are a bit deeper to hold more food, and they're made from a soft plastic that can't hurt your cat's teeth.

If your cat is having trouble eating, your vet may suggest the insertion of a feeding tube. I declined one for Isabel as I felt that she was in her last couple of years. Also, she ate tons of food anyway—it was actually her illness that sped up her metabolism and made her anorexic. Also, sometimes she'd vomit up her food so a feeding tube would have no effect on that. You'll have to discuss this possibility with your vet and decide what's the best thing to do.

VII. Managing Litter Box and Incontinence

If your cat can barely walk more than a few feet, I suggest placing her litter box within reach of her kitty bed and dishes. See the diagram in III. Setting Up A Kitty Care Station. You should place a mat or something underneath to collect any stray litter. I don't recommend using a vacuum near the kitty care station as the noise will frighten your sick cat.

Even if cats are in their end stages of life, they still want a clean and tidy living space. They'll do their best to use their litter box. This is the time to toss that tall, automated, covered contraption with steps. Get your cat a smaller kitten box, one that has lowered sides. If your cat has trouble climbing over the edge to get in, cut one side out, or buy a boot tray with short sides, or some other type of plastic container that is waterproof but can hold litter.

If your cat has reached the point where she can't get to the box, you can actually buy diapers for cats. It seems a bit silly, and even embarrassing, but you do what you have to do to care for your pet. This is also the perfect solution if your pet will recover from their illness, as it's only temporary. But even if you're managing her accidents when she's 20 years old, do let the veterinarian know that she is now experiencing incontinence.

You can use special kitty wipes to clean their bottoms and fur. It's a lot messier than you think, even though you may choose to use a washcloth to clean their faces or backs. Don't forget to wipe down their paws too. Generally, cats who reach this point won't try to wrestle with you. If they do, you'll have to wrap a towel around them, or enlist the aid of another family member.

If your cat is having trouble eliminating, or her urine or stools look abnormal, ask their vet for advice.

You'll eventually get into a regular cat care routine and it'll become second nature. You may even enjoy the process of looking after your cat, and how she needs even more love and attention from you than ever before. Please enjoy the time you spend with your cat. The next set of chapters focus on your own mental well-being and care.

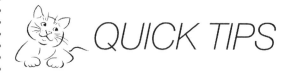

QUICK TIPS

- Set a routine for you and your cat.
- Keep your cat's mind active with play.
- Set up a kitty care station.
- Gently clean your cat with a damp cloth.
- It's simpler to give liquid medications.
- Spoon feed your cat if she's not eating.
- Use a small & basic litter box or pan.

Let the Games Begin

4. Meowing in the Streets—Living Is Celebrating

One thing I'm sure everyone can agree on is that being alive is a cause for celebration. There are many dangers inside and outside our homes, and inside our bodies that can affect our cats and us. The very nature of life is a reason for living.

It's important to take a step back and realize that being alive is a cause for celebration. Every day that you have a chronically or terminally ill cat is a day for celebration. It's like a whole new birthday each day for your pet, but instead you're celebrating them being alive for another day.

This chapter is a bit different from the one ahead about expressing appreciation. Instead, you'll be celebrating what you already have. Go ahead and decorate your cat's wet food with kitty treats, or place a kiss on their nose every morning.

Celebrating helps to encourage the positivity in your life. It may even indicate time for change or growth within yourself. You can be as smug as that expression on your cat's face as they stare at you. You've got this, and you can tackle the next challenge that comes along.

Do brag about your wonderful cat on social media. Go ahead and set up their own Facebook, Instagram, Twitter, and Pinterest accounts. Post and share regular updates about your cat. Today, they got out of bed or they ate their food. Perhaps you successfully learned how to pill them, or give them IV fluids, or solved a cat care issue that has stressed you out and stumped you for ages. Yay! You did it!

These are things that you can't take for granted, as they don't always happen, right?

This is also a good time to start taking photographs of all the cute things your cat does. Don't worry if they don't play anymore, or aren't interested in looking out the window. Snap photos of them sleeping or lying in bed. Take pics of their jellybeans or their cupcakes. Take a pic of their fluffy cat butts. If it's a cat part, it's cute!

Always remember your kitty achievements and the good times. Think back on some fun times you had with your cat. They can still continue. You'll find other tips in this book on how to spend time with your cat, but always keep it light and silly.

A day ahead of time, think up fun ways to celebrate the next day of your cat's life. Perhaps you want to cook up some chicken for them. Maybe you'll knit them a new kitty blanket and you'll wrap it up, then present it to them. Make a big deal of it, and tear the package open in front of your cat—they probably won't care much until they get to try it out—then it'll be all purrs.

Every morning jump out of bed with new purpose and happiness. You get to see your kitty again—and if they actually woke you up—then hooray! You may even wish to set the alarm a bit earlier for the next morning, and go to bed just a bit later. This will give you some extra time to get things done.

Since you're celebrating, there's nothing wrong with having a glass of wine when you're out on the weekend, or buying yourself new socks or a cat mug. Spoil yourself every now and then.

Turn your home environment into a visual party atmosphere. You may want to keep the music down low, particularly if your pet is sleeping in that room. If your cat is awake, let them watch you dance around the room. It'll lift their spirits too.

Make cat bunting and hang it from the walls. Eat from your best china and put out your nice things. There's no point in keeping your best things packed up in a closet, because you can't enjoy them when you can't see them.

If you've always wanted to buy your cat something, go ahead and buy it. There's no point in waiting to buy a soft blanket for them to enjoy, or a new toy (even if they will just cuddle with it).

Consider allowing others to join in your celebration. Have a party for your cat now, rather than a celebration of life when they're gone. Make cute kitty cupcakes and be certain you make a special treat for them too. Decorate your living room with silly cat decorations.

You can even celebrate life by doing something differently. Show up for work with a smile on your face and no makeup. Seriously, no one will notice you didn't do your makeup today, and in fact, they may wonder why you look so attractive.

Walk around in the grass in your bare feet and really notice how cool and soft the grass feels. Leave your hair down for a change. Order that dessert, because remember, no one is getting out of here alive.

Attitude is everything when you celebrate life. Once you get our of your dreary routine you'll remember what life is all about. Get out there and have some fun with your cat, right meow!

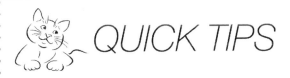 QUICK TIPS

- **Every day is a celebration with your cat.**

- **Dress up and show up for life.**

- **Have fun with your cat.**

- **Enjoy the simple things that surround you.**

5. Meow Meow Meow—Ask for Help Like a Cat

If you're reading this book, you've already asked for help. You've started by buying my book. There are many other ways to ask for help too.

Some people will enjoy the time spent looking after their sick or ailing cats, while others may find it an extremely stressful experience. If you have children, you're probably used to looking after them throughout all hours of the night when they get sick, or when they're just plain full of mischief.

You may even have dogs or other small animals that you've had to look after during some point in your life. If you've managed to figure out how to look after them, then kudos to you. But in some respects, looking after a cat can be different.

A cat can develop a shrill, high-pitched crying sound when they're in pain or distressed. They can pace the floor and constantly jump on and off the bed. They may even bat your face, or swat your arm to try and get your attention. Sure, it's cute when you're awake and playing with them, but not so great when you're trying to sleep!

If you don't have children and are used to sleeping a solid eight to nine hours a night, then it's going to be difficult making the transition to losing sleep to look after your sick cat. This is one of the harder aspects of cat care that I had to conquer.

Isabel would have cried for hours if I hadn't addressed her needs. I finally figured out, about a year in, to simply pick her up and make her comfortable on a soft blanket or her kitty pillow, then place her on my bed. I'd then turn out the light, wrap myself around her kitty bed, and gently stroke her head. She'd start purring and soon we'd both fall asleep.

I also had to ask the vet about a long-term painkiller medication. While the vet advised me on specific times of the day to give the cat her meds, I asked if I could give them at 11 am and 11 pm each night instead. The vet told me to do what I had to do. In fact, making your cat more comfortable in the morning and right before bed are two key times in your cat's daily life. It was tricky getting to a point where we both began sleeping through most of the night.

But if you ever feel stressed out or suffer insomnia, don't be afraid to ask for help. Your cat may ask for help by batting your arm or meowing loudly, or they may not ask for help at all and hide under the bed.

If you have a partner in life, you must share your difficulties with them. Just like with a sick child, the burden of responsibility for your cat shouldn't be placed on one family member. Everyone has to get up and go to work or school in the morning. If you work from home, it doesn't matter that you're at home, you still have to work!

You'll need to sit down and talk to your spouse, partner, boyfriend, girlfriend, or roommates, and work out a good schedule that suits both of you. Just like looking after baby and taking turns in the middle of the night when they cry, you can do the same for the cat.

You may also wish to have a "family meeting" and include your children. They should know that kitty is sick and mustn't be let outside. Kids naturally like to imitate us. Assign them some chores for them to do. Have them scoop the box if it needs to be done, or keep the cat's water dish clean and full. Let them smooth out kitty's blankets and kitty bed. They can also keep an eye on the cat to be certain that she is acting the same as she has been, and that her condition hasn't worsened.

The children will love to help in looking after your pets. Hey, it may even inspire them to become a veterinarian when they're ready to enter university!

You may need to share your experiences with your boss or coworkers. They care about you too, and want to know what's going on in life that has you drinking three cups of coffee in the morning and sometimes crying at your desk.

They also need to know if you need time off to attend vet visits, or just have a day off to sleep. It's best to keep them in the loop, because otherwise, they'll invent some crazy story about your life, which you wish you were in now.

Even though you're likely taking your cat to the clinic regularly, whether it's for checkups, to have injections, or IV fluids done, you may forget that your cat's vet is also there to provide assistance with the tough stuff.

You can ask the vet what they suggest for getting your pet to sleep through the night, or what to do if they skip the litter box, or are difficult to pill. Remember that the vet can't tell you all the things all the time, so you must be specific and ask questions. If they don't know, they can direct you to the right place, or they can order in products that can aid you in your cat care duties.

Don't forget about your own doctor. During this stressful time you should look after yourself too. It may be time to have a regular checkup and have lab tests done. Some of the most common nutritional deficiencies of stressed-out people are usually with the B-vitamins. They can also give you a Vitamin B12 injection if you're lacking. Anemia, or the lack of iron in your blood, can also be a concern, particularly if you're not eating right, or skipping meals. If you feel extra tired, even though you lose only one or two hours of sleep a night, do book a doctor's appointment.

Besides our physical care, our mental, emotional, and psychological well-being can be at stake too. But remember that it's only temporary, until your cat gets better or passes away. I'd avoid taking anti-depressants, as most people who take them report that they aren't good for the long term.

Seek other ways of feeling better—head outdoors to sit in the sun, take vitamins and supplements, eat berries, eat more protein and citrus fruits, nuts, and oatmeal. Book an appointment at the salon to get a nice back and shoulder massage, and mani-pedi. Try aromatherapy to make you feel better. There are even some essential oils that are safe to use around your cat (but please research first), and you'll both feel better!

If there is someone in your life who is going through something similar, then reach out to them and see if you can provide mutual support to each other.

If you have a best friend, keep them in the loop about what's going on in your life. Be sure to ask them about their life too, so it's not all about you.

Did you know that many people don't have best friends? Often their spouses or cats are their best friends. But you don't have to chat with a best friend to make yourself feel better. It doesn't even have to be an ongoing friendship. Short conversations are good too. Let the cashier at the store know you're stressed out about your cat. They'll provide you with a smile and warm wishes.

There are also dozens of online forums and social media groups you can join to talk about your cat, or the health of your cat. Don't be afraid to post and ask for help. There are hundreds of people online who want to offer their help and advice—just take some of it with a grain of salt, and don't be afraid to block anyone abusive.

You can also hire cat sitters who can come to your home during the day and give kitty her medication or fluids, or just check on her.

Did you know there are catcams? This is a device that you set up on the floor. You can have a one-way or a two-way video conversation with your cat. Some can even shoot treats out so your cat comes rushing when it turns on. There are even devices that allow you to call your cat to talk to them on the phone.

Often you may experience separation anxiety from your cat while you're at work. These devices can help in a way, because they help you to stay in touch with your cat.

There are also meal subscription services that prepare your food in advance. You open up the package, toss it into the pan or the oven, and then cook it. It makes preparing meals much simpler, and can actually give you an extra hour per day to spend time with kitty.

Often it's the little things that can help to make you feel better. Try to think up clever ways to look after your cat or yourself. Most likely by now you'll have a few ideas to jot down on paper. If you need help, then ask for it like a cat.

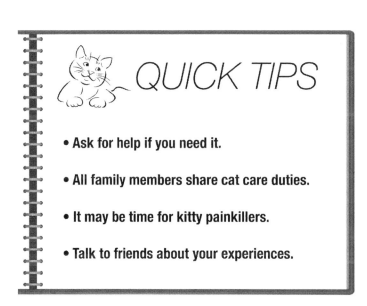

QUICK TIPS

- Ask for help if you need it.

- All family members share cat care duties.

- It may be time for kitty painkillers.

- Talk to friends about your experiences.

6. Purring Makes the World Go Round—Caring for You

Even though your fur family is going to be the most important part of your world, you're also 100% important too. You must always care for you, even when you're undergoing stress. Did you know that the stress you endure when looking after a sick pet is exactly the same as the caregiver stress of people who look after sick or aging parents? Often the major concern is that people start mourning the loss of their loved ones before they're gone.

This is not only ridiculous—no one knows how much time we have left—but it defeats the purpose of life. And your cat is certainly not going to want you to feel sad or unhappy.

Unfortunately, this type of caregiver stress is unavoidable, but the good news is that it's also manageable. Some people manage it better than others, otherwise no one would have children. But unlike our regular jobs where we can take off a week or four to hang out at the beach, we can't do that when we're looking after a sick cat.

In fact, many professional cat sitters or cat boarding businesses won't accept pets when they're extremely sick. Your vet may take your pet in, at a rate of hundreds of dollars per day. So, until you feel that you can trust someone else with the care of your sick pet, it's unlikely that you're going to get away for a vacation.

The best way to manage stress is to decrease its impact on your body. This means you're going to need to take small breaks throughout the day.

You want to always keep on breathing and never hold your breath. Your body needs a good amount of oxygen in its blood so it can keep you going. When you take a few good deep breaths in, it will help to instantly relax you. Avoid shallow breathing as it places your body in a heightened state of stress.

One of my favourite breathing techniques is called the box technique. It's simple and easy to learn. Remember that a box has four sides. To begin, breathe in for four seconds, then hold your breath for four seconds. Take the next four seconds to breathe out. Then hold for four seconds. Get it? Four by four by four by four?

Visualization techniques can help you too. All you have to do is imagine yourself in a calm and relaxing environment. It may be on a beach somewhere, or a cruise ship where you're sipping a nice rum drink.

Many people like to have a nice massage. If you can't get away to the salon or massage therapy clinic, do it yourself. They have back massagers and rollers that you can buy from any store that sells healthcare products. You can also use your hands to massage the parts of your shoulders and back that you can reach.

If you have a special-needs washroom at work, lock the door and rub your back against that handlebar beside the toilet.

Maybe you can even train your cat to jump on your back and make biscuits!

Have you ever forced yourself to smile? Did you notice how it made you feel better? Try it the next time you feel sad and depressed. In fact, smiling at the most inappropriate times is going to make you feel so silly and stupid that that alone will bring a smile to your face! Plus, your cat loves it when you smile, so go ahead and smile at her right meow.

If you are religious, you may pray. But even if you don't, you can say little mantras to yourself. You can even sing them to your cat. I had at least a series of 20 different little songs I'd sing to Isabel out loud, or to myself in my head.

Here are just a few suggestions:

• I've got this.
• I love my kitty cat.
• Today is a happy day.
• One paw two paw three paw four.
• You're my kitty cat how I love that.

Whenever you feel stressed or anxious, sing your mantra out loud at least ten times. If you're out in public, sing it in your head.

Avoid asking why this is happening to you. Many other people have healthy cats, right? Well, not exactly. Many people keep bad things bottled up in their bodies. But you shouldn't keep them bottled up. All of our emotions are a natural part of life.

Meditation and journalling are always recommended for people who are finding it difficult in getting through life. There is plenty of advice online for various meditation techniques, so I won't go through them here. As for journalling, buy yourself the cutest kitty cat notebook you can find and start writing stuff down. Get your feelings out of your head and onto paper. The best time is about two hours before bed, so you can clear your mind and be ready for sleep.

You may also wish to write some questions in your journal, such as finding a better way to dose your cat with meds, or how to trim their claws without them giving you a kitty smackdown. Then the next day this will give you something to figure out when you're tired of your usual work.

Some people like to count to 10, or count backwards from 100. This helps you to achieve mindfulness and stay in the moment, rather than your mind wandering off on a tangent that you can't solve.

It may help if you think up funny stories about your cat. Today, she stole your wallet and bought herself the most expensive cat castle online, or she danced around the neighbour's dog. They're kind of silly but should make you smile. You can even draw photos and share them online if you want.

Exercise, yoga, and just plain stretching is also good for your body. Or, get outside and walk around the block.

Everyone has time to do that. Some people may even shake their hands out or jump up and down. Whatever works for you. No matter what you do, changing your routine and getting up and moving around will help your lungs to breathe easier so you feel better.

Aromatherapy can also be beneficial, but just be certain to choose essential oils that you aren't allergic to and that are safe around your cat. There is plenty of info online about cat-safe essential oils that I won't cover here. Aromatherapy is particularly beneficial to the senses, and can help you to calm down and breathe easier. You can simply place a few drops of essential oil in a small ceramic dish in your room. Do keep it away from your cat just in case they like to lick things they shouldn't.

I don't advise burning candles or using plug-ins around a sick cat, plus, you will be too busy to keep an eye on them. Simply pour a few drops of essential oil into a small dish and store it on a shelf away from the reach of pets.

It's important to keep up with pampering you. A nice hot soak at the end of a long day with some nice lavender-scented bubblebath will help you to sleep better at night. Did you know that Calgon is still around? Yes, and you can buy bath bombs and powdered bath softeners too.

Don't forget about the power of music, but don't turn it up too loud. Even some nice classical music, or nature music, is also good for your cat. Play some lively music on occasion and get up and dance.

Sometimes you just need to have a good cry. The best way to tackle this is during pre-scheduled time. Promise yourself that when you're on a break at work, or when you're at home and your cat is having a nap, to slip away to the bathroom and cry for five minutes. Crying releases natural endorphins to make you feel good afterwards. You can't stop yourself from crying so you might as well go for it.

It can be difficult to keep up with regular meals when you have your cat on a strict schedule of syringe feeding, fluids, medications, and cleaning, but it's important to stick with your daily three. Don't skip meals. If you must eat a TV dinner every now and then, add some carrot sticks or grapes to your meal. At least you'll still be getting some fresh nutrients.

There's no point in self-pity or asking why things happened the way they did. Simply become a fighter and accept that illness and disease are also a part of life, just as death is at the end. Read through some of the advice in this chapter when you feel down. It'll help you to stay in better control and feel much happier. Take the time you need to get things done.

Don't be afraid to tell friends, family, or colleagues, that no, you don't have time to do this or that because you're doing something that matters to you. Is it really necessary to sign up for classes after work? It may be time to take a break, at least until kitty is stabilized and can be left alone for longer periods of time.

Remember to always take care of you.

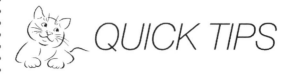

QUICK TIPS

- Don't forget to look after yourself too.

- Never grieve for a cat who's still alive.

- Schedule small breaks.

- Put a smile on your face.

May the Odds Be Ever in Your Flavour

7. Getting Into Catnip—Completing Your Kitty Bucket List

Creating a bucket list for you and your cat will not only be fun, but you'll have a lifetime of memories. There will come a time when the pain and remorse of your cat's passing will turn to one of blessing and enjoyment. You'll be able to brag to your new kitty about how their predecessor played a wonderful role in your life.

Some people may be uncertain what exactly a bucket list can be. Usually it's something that humans do for themselves. A bucket list for humans is when you figure out what you'd like to do before you die, and you write it down as a commitment for the future. It's a number of experiences or achievements that a person hopes to have or accomplish during their lifetime.

They're kind of like goals, but more of a "must-do list" then something you attempt to achieve, such as taking a trip to Egypt or hitting it big in the lottery. In other words, they should be things that are more easily attainable, otherwise, you're going to be in for heartbreak.

Just like with your own bucket list, a kitty bucket list consists of things you can do with your cat before he or she dies. You'd be surprised at how many pets pass on and their humans don't even have any photographs or videos of them! If this has ever happened to you, hopefully another family member at least had a photo or two on their Facebook page. And if you had photos but misplaced them, check on

Facebook, as you may have posted the photos on there. They won't be hi-res, but who cares? Your friends may also have photos or videos if they've ever been over to your place.

After my Cristobel passed away I found over 1200 photographs of her on my computer, and even a few printed copies in my desk. I had no regrets there, and can still look at her in photographs and videos whenever I want.

So, just how do you create a kitty bucket list?

- Begin by making a list of things to do with your cat. These are just suggestions. You may think up many more on your own.

- Take photographs of your cat with their favourite toys, kitty beds, or in sleeping areas.

- Snap a photo of your cat doing a favourite trick.

- Take photos of your beloved pet in their favourite spots around the home.

- Take a selfie when your pet is sitting on your lap.

- If your cat does anything unique or silly, record a video.

- Your digital camera may have a video setting, or use your smart phone or tablet to do it.

- Order a custom sterling silver necklace of your cat's image that has been etched onto the surface. These are usually under $80.

- Order a custom stuffie of your cat. These can be extremely expensive, over $300+, but can be a wonderful memorial after they're gone.

- Use the audio-record function on your phone, computer, or tablet and record your cat purring or meowing.

- Put your cat on a harness and leash and take them outside for a walk, or around the outside of your home.

- Hire a professional photographer to come to your home and take a family photo with the entire family, including all humans and pets.

- Take your cat to the Santa photo session at your local pet store in December.

- Play kitty dress-up and take photos of your cat wearing cute outfits and accessories.

- Grab a laser toy or ribbon toy and actually play with your cat.

- Have a kitty salon day. This involves a good brushing, wiping down dirty regions with kitty shampoo, trimming claws, and cleaning ears with cotton puffs.

- Give your cat some catnip and have the camera ready!

- Set a channel to a nature program and move your kitty's perch in front of the TV to let them enjoy some entertainment.

- Download soothing classical music and set it to play for everyone's enjoyment.

- Have a puppet show. Grab your cat's toys and create a little play for them.

- Drop what you're doing and simply sit with your cat for an hour to appreciate how they've made your life so much better.

- Take a moment and smile at your cat.

- Have a conversation with your cat. Try meowing back at them, or even doing silent meows.

- Put kitty perches around your home so your cat can watch you while you work, watch TV, cook, etc.

- Buy a photo album and have your kitty's photographs printed out at Walmart or London Drugs. Put them in a photo album.

- Buy a kitty scrapbook and start filling in the questions about your cat. Write little stories and paste in photographs. Some even have sections for vet records.

- When you find stray whiskers around the house, tuck them into a ziplock bag and place them in your kitty scrapbook.

- Take fur clippings of your pet and use a glue gun or tape to secure them into your cat's photo album.

- Keep your kitty's claw sheaths and store them in a ziplock bag.

- Keep cat food labels and put them in the album.

- Buy a nice large decorative box and store your cat's old things in them.

- If you live in a small home and feel you can't keep your cat's old things, grab the camera and take photographs. It's the next best thing, and you can look up their old stuff anytime you want.

- Add your own ideas here!

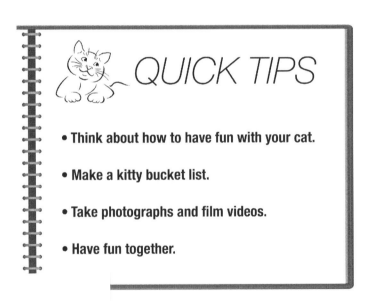

QUICK TIPS

- **Think about how to have fun with your cat.**

- **Make a kitty bucket list.**

- **Take photographs and film videos.**

- **Have fun together.**

8. Expurrressing Gratitude—Appreciate What Mew Have

When you're stressed out after looking after a sick cat, you may experience feelings of despair and depression. The only way to cope is to reverse your feelings. Just how do some people stay happy, even when life is tossing cat poop in their face? Most likely they've learned how to expurress gratitude.

This means appreciating what you have, not what you don't have. Sure, we all want to fly with our cats on private jumbo jets where they're served catviar while we get champagne, but the reality is that most of us won't get to do these things.

Strangely, our busy lifestyles seem to focus on what we don't have, rather than what we do. Television, film, magazines, and newspapers are all to blame for that. Even listening to our neighbours, coworkers, friends, and family sometimes—it seems like no one is happy with their place in life. Everyone focusses on what they don't have.

So, let's change that around. The first thing you should know is that your kitty is here right meow. They may no longer be kittens, bursting full of energy, or eating all their food—but who cares? They're alive and that's all that matters.

It helps to count your blessings. Just what do you have in life right meow? A furry little companion who loves you a lot. You may need to write reminders in a little journal with a cute cat on the front. Place it on your desk and write in it each day. Go back and read through your thoughts.

Sometimes it helps to gain perspective by heading outdoors. The Japanese have an ancient practice called "tree bathing". Basically, you grab a blanket and go and sit under a tree for an hour. You set aside your electronics. You can do crafts or read a book if you wish, but it's important to tune out the world and listen to nature.

Spend time learning how to be in the moment. When you're with your cat, don't fantasize about them being better. Appreciate them for who they are now. Yes, they're sick, and maybe they can't get out of bed. But that's all right, it's a natural part of the healing process and the process of life.

Gently pet and stroke your pet and give them a kiss. Hang around with them and listen to the sounds they hear. It's important to stop comparing you or your cat to other owners or their pets. Their situations are not applicable to you. As we said in the

"Platitudes, Catitudes" chapter, sometimes you must tune out what people say to you.

You may have to downsize your life and your home for your cat. So what? You're the only one keeping track anyway. Yes, you might have to sell electronics or jewellery to cover those vet bills, but the most precious object in your life is your pet. And remember what I said in a prior chapter—take photos of the things you treasure before they're gone.

So, now you have a simpler lifestyle with your cat. You can no longer go to the bar each night, or see a play every Saturday night. One day you'll do those things again, but for now you have a wonderful cat who needs your time.

Always ask questions. How can you make your situation better? How can you make the life of your cat better? Often it's something little and the answer may be right in front of you. Maybe your cat would be more comfortable with a heating pad designed for cats. These have auto shutoffs in case you forget. Many cats who experience pain would love heat on their arthritic joints. Or, perhaps your cat is annoyed by the dog. Relocating your cat's bed to the bedroom and shutting the door may help.

You also need to let go of hatred, anger, and other

negative thoughts. By now you've experienced them, and they only made you feel worse. It's time to put them in a box and store them away. You don't have the time or energy to dwell on these negative thoughts. Do a mental let-go of that box. You need to forgive nature, god, or whatever you believe in for giving your cat this illness. This is an important part of the healing process.

Always remember to smile even if you don't feel like it. Some people like to tie a ribbon around their wrist to remind them of such things. Be sure to smile at your cat often. They can pick up and sense your moods. If they see you smiling, it will make them feel better. You'll both worry less about the situation.

Go and stand in front of a mirror for 20 minutes a day and smile at yourself. Set a timer. Some people stick a pencil between their lips to hold that smile in position. As you smile, think about all the good things that have come your way.

What unique things have you experienced in yours and your cat's life that no one else has? Does your cat do cute things? Do they do tricks or meow in an amusing way? Do this while you practice your mirror smiles.

Do you have beliefs, faiths, or a religion? You may

wish to focus on the positivity of these beliefs too. They can give you hope to go on.

Besides a journal, some people like to create little notes about something they've been grateful for in their day. Then they toss them into a nice bottle or vase. At the end of the month they dump them out and read through them. There are also other ways to create gratitude boxes—use your creativity.

Allow your family to join in with expressing gratitude. Have people go around the table and think up something specific to your cat being a part of your family. Often you'll be surprised at the sentiments. You may also wish to record these in your journal.

What was something funny that your cat did today? Were they extra cute? Did they do something amusing but very bad? Make a note of it in your journal.

Don't forget to thank your cat for being in your life. Give them a little pet, give them a kiss. Tell them how much you love them when you wake up in the morning, or when you go to bed at night.

You may wish to save some of your gratitude for bedtime. Keep your journal or your gratitude vase by your bed. You'll go to sleep much easier thinking positive thoughts, instead of worrying about how sick your kitty is.

Always remember to show up in the morning and be present. Your kitty is depending on you. When you're happy and aware, they'll feel more comforted, which just may give them an edge they need to heal up and get better!

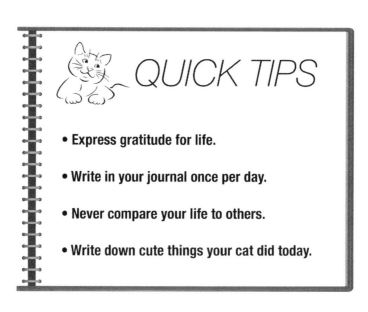

QUICK TIPS

- Express gratitude for life.

- Write in your journal once per day.

- Never compare your life to others.

- Write down cute things your cat did today.

9. Purring Among the Stars—What Happens Next?

As much as we fantasize about our cats being with us for our entire lives, sadly, our beloved pets don't live as long as we do. With the average cat age being 12 to 14 years old before they pass, that means that we must open up our hearts to several different cats in our lifetimes.

If your cat has passed, then it's one of the most stressful moments of your life. Back in 2009, I did an internship at a psychiatrist's office. It was the end of the day and I had a chat with the doctor there. I was telling him how I'd lost my beloved Cristobel, and how hard a time I'd had in dealing with her death.

The psychiatrist had told me that these were normal feelings, and that often people grieved their dead pets to a level much deeper than losing a parent. I have lost both my parents, and this was truth—losing my cats was far more difficult. I was so glad that a professional had validated my feelings, and that I wasn't doing anything wrong!

There are five things that happen after your cat has passed.

Physical Effects—You may experience headaches, dizziness, nausea, insomnia, shortness of breath, panic attacks, and other health issues.

Intellectual Effects—You feel like you're in an unreal world. Some people experience hallucinations. Time may pass by too slowly or too quickly.

Emotional Effects—You may experience feelings of depression, sadness, anxiety, irritability, and even anger. You want to blame others. You may feel life is out of your control and you're helpless as a result.

Social Effects—You may experience feelings of isolation as you're stuck at home caring for kitty. After kitty is gone, you'll feel your friends have left you, as you're still all alone.

Spiritual Effects—You may have doubts about God or Mother Nature who would allow you and your pet to suffer. You may try bargaining with them or praying.

Many people may wonder what they should do after their cat has died. Sometimes your cat passes at the vet, as you feel "it's time" and that they are suffering too much. Your vet will assist you through the process and help you to make arrangements.

Sometimes you decide you want your pet to die naturally, so you look after them to their end of days. Your cat may have cried out for your attention, so you went to her—this is what happened minutes before Isabel passed—and sometimes you find them in their bed the next morning, having passed quietly away.

You may wrap a blanket around their precious body, and wait until the sun rises and your closest vet clinic opens. Most vet clinics will accept deceased cats. You don't need to visit your own clinic, particularly if it's far away.

Some people think they must place their pet in the fridge or freezer. I don't advise that, for two reasons. One is due to hygienic reasons; the second is that it's your beloved, and would you do that to your spouse or child? Simply place a plastic bag under them, wrap a blanket around them, leaving their face free, and wait until morning. Yes, the body may smell a bit, but it's no worse than meat gone bad. Death is a natural process and not something that should ever horrify or disgust you. I advise against keeping the body outdoors, due to pests and other animals.

Once you've booked your appointment in the morning, bring your pet to the vet. Once there, you can make arrangements.

You have three options for dealing with your cat's remains. One is to leave your cat at home, and bury them in the backyard. You may want to be aware of city utilities before you do that though, as you want your pet buried far enough down that no animal can dig them out. You may wish to place your cat in a box first. If you go this route, be sure you're going to stick around for many years, or be aware you'll have to leave your pet there if you do move, or that your pet may be dug up if there's ever a redevelopment.

The second option involves a public burial. This is where your cat is buried in a public space with many other pets. This is a cheap alternative for people who don't have a lot of cash. But you won't know where the location is, nor will you be able to visit.

The third alternative is to have a private burial. This involves the cremation of your cat. You'll receive the cremains in about two weeks' time. These are contained within an urn. You may choose what type of urn you want. You can even move them into a different urn at a later date. The urn can have a name, date, and words engraved onto a little plaque. You may choose to keep the urn on your mantelpiece or shelf at home, or bury them in the backyard. Many people choose to have their pets' remains buried with them when they pass.

You may also wish to have a paw impression or paw prints made of your cat's paws. I had one done of Isabel. People think they're cute! You can choose size, one or both paws, and different colours.

If you forgot to take fur snips earlier, you can do this now.

There's no right way or wrong way when you decide what happens next. These are your choices. Do what feels right to you, and what comforts you best.

It's going to be difficult to keep on going when you're missing your beloved cat. When they were sick you likely had to rearrange your entire life to adjust to caring for them. Then they're gone, and suddenly, your routine changes again.

How odd and puzzling that suddenly your life becomes much simpler and easier—yet you're horrendously depressed! This is why the person who constantly has bad things happen to them can be the happiest person on the planet, while a millionaire can be chronically depressed—it's more of perception of what is normal in life and choosing your own path.

According to Elizabeth Kubler-Ross, who wrote the world-renowned book "On Death and Dying", there are five stages for grief. You may go through one or all of them, or go backwards or forwards. You can find more information online for this process, or read her book if you wish.

I invite you to go back and reread Chapters 5. Meow Meow Meow—Ask for Help Like a Cat; 6. Purring Makes the World Go Round—Caring for You; and 8. Expurressing Gratitude—Appreciate What Mew Have. You'll just have to adjust them to your own current situation.

Be happy and proud in knowing that you made a difference in your cat's life. Remember how your cat stared at you with that smug expression on their face? They were happy that you were their human, if only for a few years in the lifetime of this wonderful universe that we live in right meow.

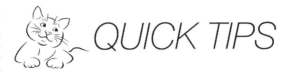 *QUICK TIPS*

- Death is that final natural stage to life.

- Find a grief counsellor if you need to talk.

- Celebrate your cat's life with memorabilia.

- Be proud of your role in your cat's life.

Conclusion—One Final Meow

Thank you for letting me share my journey for you. It's been a long hard journey, full of litter boxes and sometimes just a bit too much cat fur. By now you should have a better understanding and acceptance of your own sick, chronically ill, or terminally ill cat.

I wish you the best of luck in continuing on with your journey, as likely your kitty has made it this far, whereas I lost my Isabel before I had even finished this book.

I hope that some of my cat care tips have given you some ideas to help you look after your own cat. I know not all of them work for all cats—each kitty is a wondpurrful individual —but hopefully you can try some of them and think up even more that will work for you and your cat's life.

Always remember that if your cat's condition changes for the worse, to bring them to the veterinarian to have it checked out. It might just be a part of that process that we'll all eventually go through, but in many instances, there is something that can be done to make your cat more comfortable.

Remember to always show up (for life), put in your best effort, and give your cat a kiss, pet, or three throughout the day.

I hope you'll check out my Photo Gallery at the end of the book, look up some of the Resources I've provided, and like and follow me on Facebook and your other favourite social media channels.

Please stay in touch and post a review on your favourite review site when you have time. I do hope you feel much better about life and can purr along with the rest of us right meow.

Happy Purring!
Melanie Dixon

Photo Gallery—Isabel

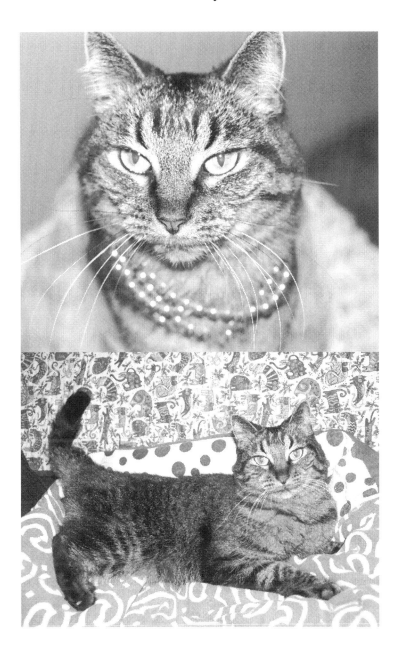

Photo Gallery—Cristobel

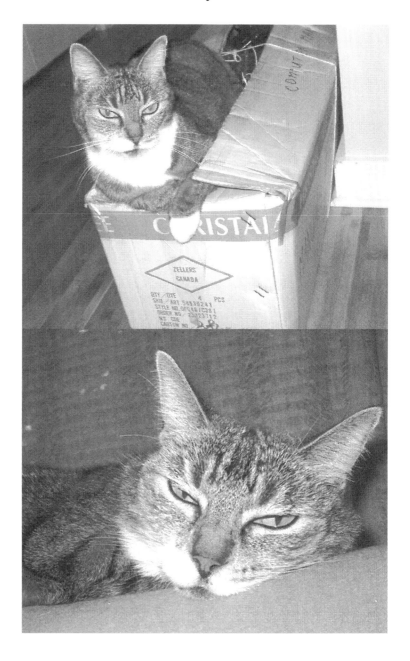

Helpful Kitty Care Resources

The following resources may provide you some additional support when you need help with caring for your beloved kitty. These sites provide free information online. But if your kitty is healthy and happy, I highly recommend that you get one of the pet insurance plans for them ASAP. If they ever suffer an accident, or get sick, then your costs will be minimal.

For general information about the care or health of your cat:

Modern Cat Magazine: https://moderncat.com
Catster Magazine: http://www.catster.com
Pet MD: https://www.petmd.com
Canada Humane Society: https://www.cfhs.ca
Your local SPCA, ASPCA, RSPCA, or Municipal Animal Services may offer low-cost spay and neuter or emergency animal care.
Pet Parent Life Hacks: https://www.facebook.com/pethacksdodo/
Wikihow.com: Search pet articles with supportive graphics.
Facebook: Pet Loss Grief and Terminal Illness Support Group

Pet Insurance:
    https://trupanion.com
    https://www.gopetplan.ca/
    https://get.petsplusus.com
    https://www.petsecure.com
    https://www.caapets.com
    https://www.petinsurance.com

Acknowledgemeownts

Thank mew to the numerous kitties who have brightened my life in the Royal City through the past few years, including Cristobel and Isabel.

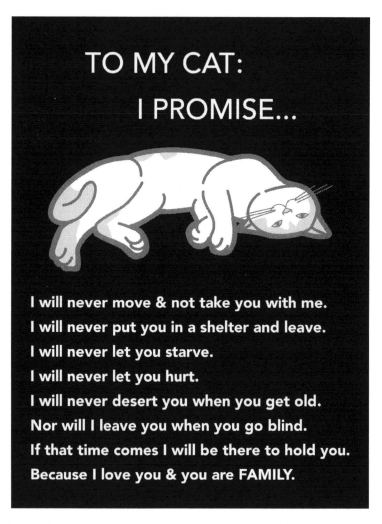

TO MY CAT:
I PROMISE...

I will never move & not take you with me.
I will never put you in a shelter and leave.
I will never let you starve.
I will never let you hurt.
I will never desert you when you get old.
Nor will I leave you when you go blind.
If that time comes I will be there to hold you.
Because I love you & you are FAMILY.

Design: Melanie Dixon | Illustration: Pixabay | Text: Unknown Cat Lover

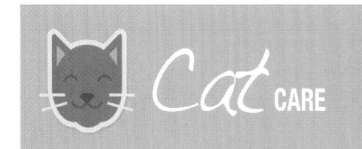

Cat CARE

DAILY MEDICATION & FEEDING SCHEDULE		MEALS & TREATS	PLAYTIME
7 AM			
8 AM			
9 AM			

DAILY MEDICATION & FEEDING SCHEDULE	
10 AM	
11 AM	
12 PM	
1 PM	
2 PM	
3 PM	
4 PM	
5 PM	
6 PM	
7 PM	
8 PM	
9 PM	
10 PM	
11 PM	

CARE NEEDS	DISCUSS WITH VET

NOTES	SHOPPING LIST

89

About the Author

For an inexplicable reason, Melanie Dixon moved into New Westminster and never left. She's a professionally published online content writer and marketer who also enjoys writing speculative fiction. Besides numerous published articles and short stories, she also has two published books: *The Aquaria Chronicles*; and *Just One More Purr: Chronic and Terminal Illness Support for Cats and the Humans Who Love Them*.

She has a degree in gemmology, and holds diplomas as a medical office assistant, graphic designer, and web designer, with various certificates in human and pet first aid, writing, and marketing.

She has short stories published in the *Confederacy of Steam Versus Zombies Anthology*, as well as in *Zombified: Hazardous Material, Devolution Z: October Issue, Antipodean Steam Guild Journal: Issue One*, and many more.

She is known for her professionally published online content writing as Mel Dawn, with over 20,000 articles scattered over the web on any good day.

She won the Telus Journalism Award in 2009 for her magazine articles in regional and provincial magazines.

Mel was a writer panelist at VCON 2014 and the Creative Ink Festivals from 2016 to 2018.

Thank Mew for Reading!

Thank you for purchasing and reading Just One More Purr: Chronic and Terminal Illness Support for Cats and the Humans Who Love Them.

If you enjoyed reading this book I'd appreciate it if you left a favourable review on your favourite review website.

Please visit my social media channels for information about upcoming book releases or promotions.

Thank mew very much!

Please follow Mel on these Social Media Channels:

Facebook: https://www.facebook.com/royalcitymel/
https://www.facebook.com/Catews19876/

Twitter: https://twitter.com/MelDawn1

Pinterest: https://www.pinterest.com/meldawn9/

Blogs: http://royalcitymel.blogspot.ca
https://meldawn9.wordpress.com

Website: https://meldawn.wixsite.com/melaniedawndixon

Goodreads: goo.gl/Od7E6Z

Your Notes

Your Cat's Vet Information

Cat's Name (s):

Name of Veterinarian:
Name of Vet Clinic:
Address:

Email Address:
Telephone Number:

Medications:

Special Treatments:

Cat Sitter Information:

Wet Food Brand:
Dry Food Brand:
Treats Brand:

Update

Hi Readers! I wrote this book over a year ago now, after an early spring 2018 release. I'm so glad that you've joined me on this journey of love, and sometimes pain.

It's been over a year since Isabel has passed away, and not a day goes by that I don't find myself missing her, and wishing she is by my side.

But I also have some good news to share with you. On April 2, 2018, I adopted a cat! She is called Pumpkin Roxy Dixon and she is 11 years old.

She is extremely affectionate and well-trained. She will "touch" for a treat, and knows how to sit, jump up, and sometimes lie down.

At first I wasn't certain if we were going to bond. She had a rough time moving in. Then one day, I realized that she may not be the cat I wanted, but she is certainly the cat I need.

Pumpkin is my therapy cat and is always there, ready for a hug, kiss, or cuddle. I look forward to caring for my Pumpkin through her senior years.

~Mel

Other Books By Melanie Dixon

Besides "Just One More Purr" I should have some other books available soon on Amazon or through email purchase.

Self-Help Care Book:
Just One More Purr

Young Adult:
Aqua Marine
Aqua Mariner
Aqua Marine Biologist
The Aquaria Chronicles

Poetry:
Zombie Poetry

Adult Horror:
Unnamed Zombie Series TBA

Photo Books:
Topper Dawn Doll Melanie
Isabel the Cat

Please contact me by email if you wish to purchase a print copy through me, or a PDF. I can do my best to provide Kindle or other book formats for eBooks too.